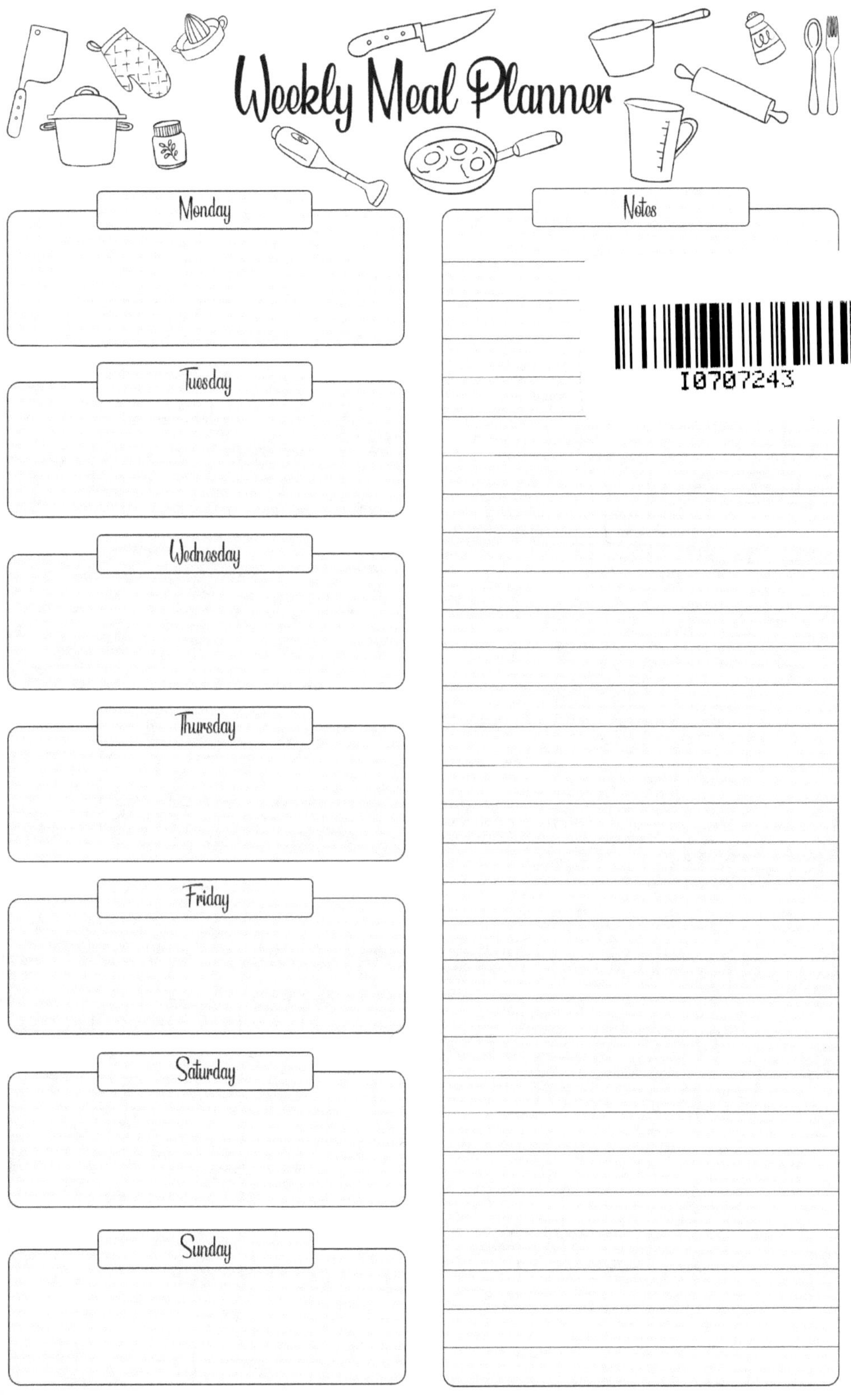

Weekly Meal Planner
Monday
Tuesday
Wednesday
Thursday
Friday
Saturday
Sunday
Notes
I0707243

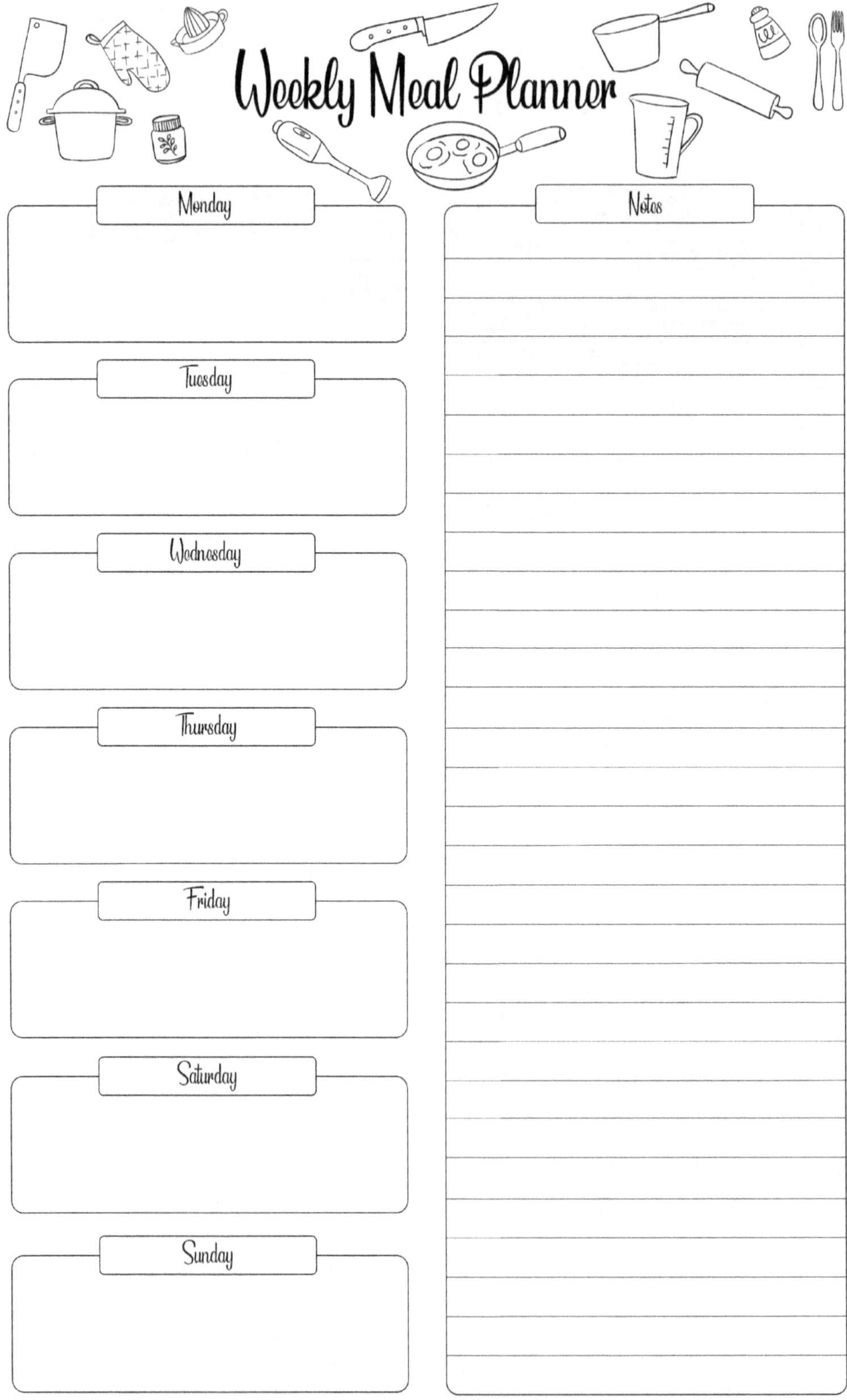

Weekly Meal Planner
Monday
Tuesday
Wednesday
Thursday
Friday
Saturday
Sunday
Notes

Weekly Meal Planner

Monday

Tuesday

Wednesday

Thursday

Friday

Saturday

Sunday

Notes

Weekly Meal Planner

Monday

Tuesday

Wednesday

Thursday

Friday

Saturday

Sunday

Notes

Weekly Meal Planner

Monday

Tuesday

Wednesday

Thursday

Friday

Saturday

Sunday

Notes

Weekly Meal Planner

Monday

Tuesday

Wednesday

Thursday

Friday

Saturday

Sunday

Notes

Weekly Meal Planner

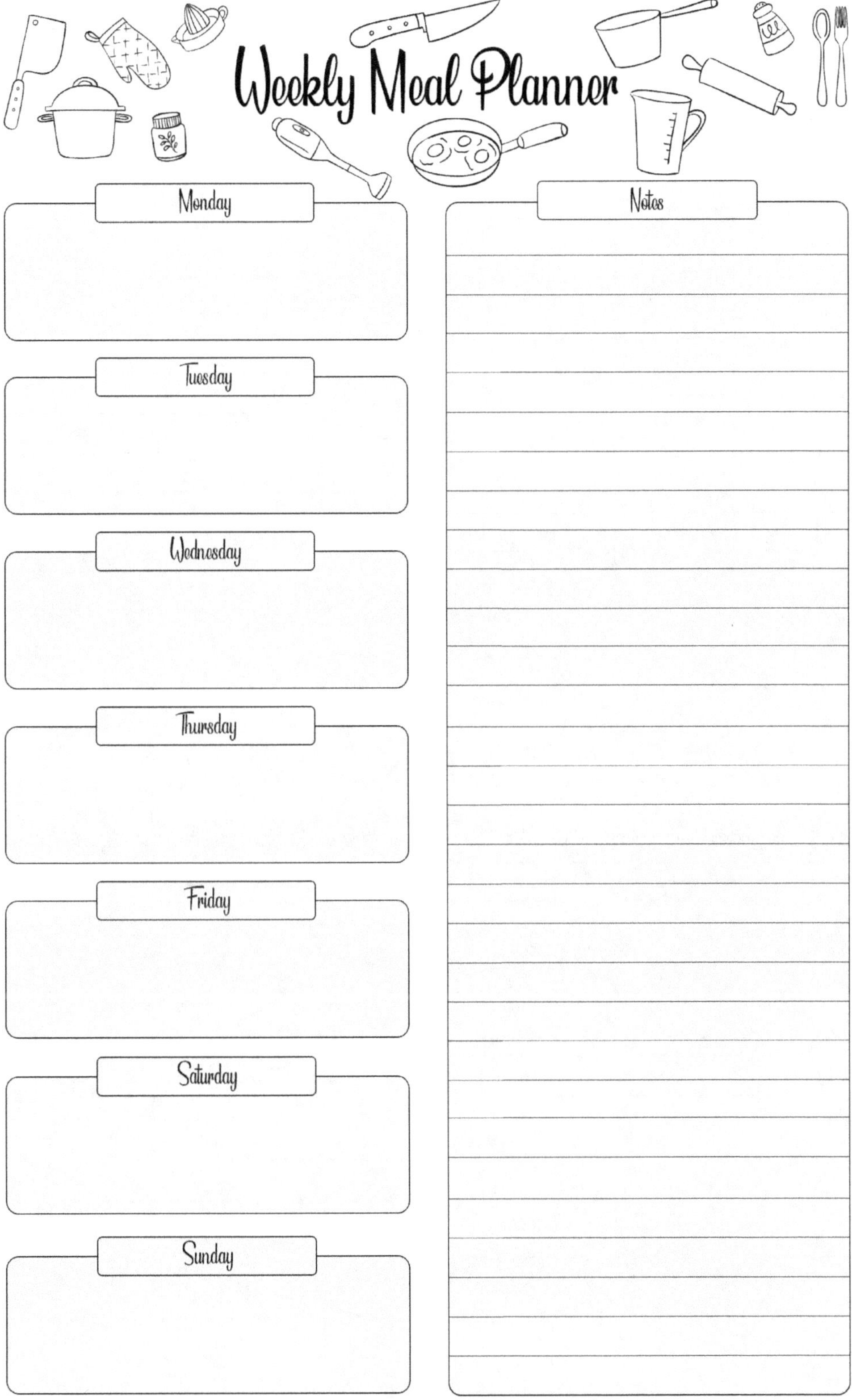

Monday

Tuesday

Wednesday

Thursday

Friday

Saturday

Sunday

Notes

Weekly Meal Planner

Monday

Tuesday

Wednesday

Thursday

Friday

Saturday

Sunday

Notes

Weekly Meal Planner

Monday

Tuesday

Wednesday

Thursday

Friday

Saturday

Sunday

Notes

Weekly Meal Planner

Monday	Notes
Tuesday	
Wednesday	
Thursday	
Friday	
Saturday	
Sunday	

Weekly Meal Planner

Monday

Tuesday

Wednesday

Thursday

Friday

Saturday

Sunday

Notes

Weekly Meal Planner

Monday

Tuesday

Wednesday

Thursday

Friday

Saturday

Sunday

Notes

Weekly Meal Planner

Monday	Notes
Tuesday	
Wednesday	
Thursday	
Friday	
Saturday	
Sunday	

Weekly Meal Planner

Monday

Tuesday

Wednesday

Thursday

Friday

Saturday

Sunday

Notes

Weekly Meal Planner

Monday

Tuesday

Wednesday

Thursday

Friday

Saturday

Sunday

Notes

Weekly Meal Planner

Monday

Tuesday

Wednesday

Thursday

Friday

Saturday

Sunday

Notes

Weekly Meal Planner

Monday

Tuesday

Wednesday

Thursday

Friday

Saturday

Sunday

Notes

Weekly Meal Planner

Monday	Notes

| Tuesday |

| Wednesday |

| Thursday |

| Friday |

| Saturday |

| Sunday |

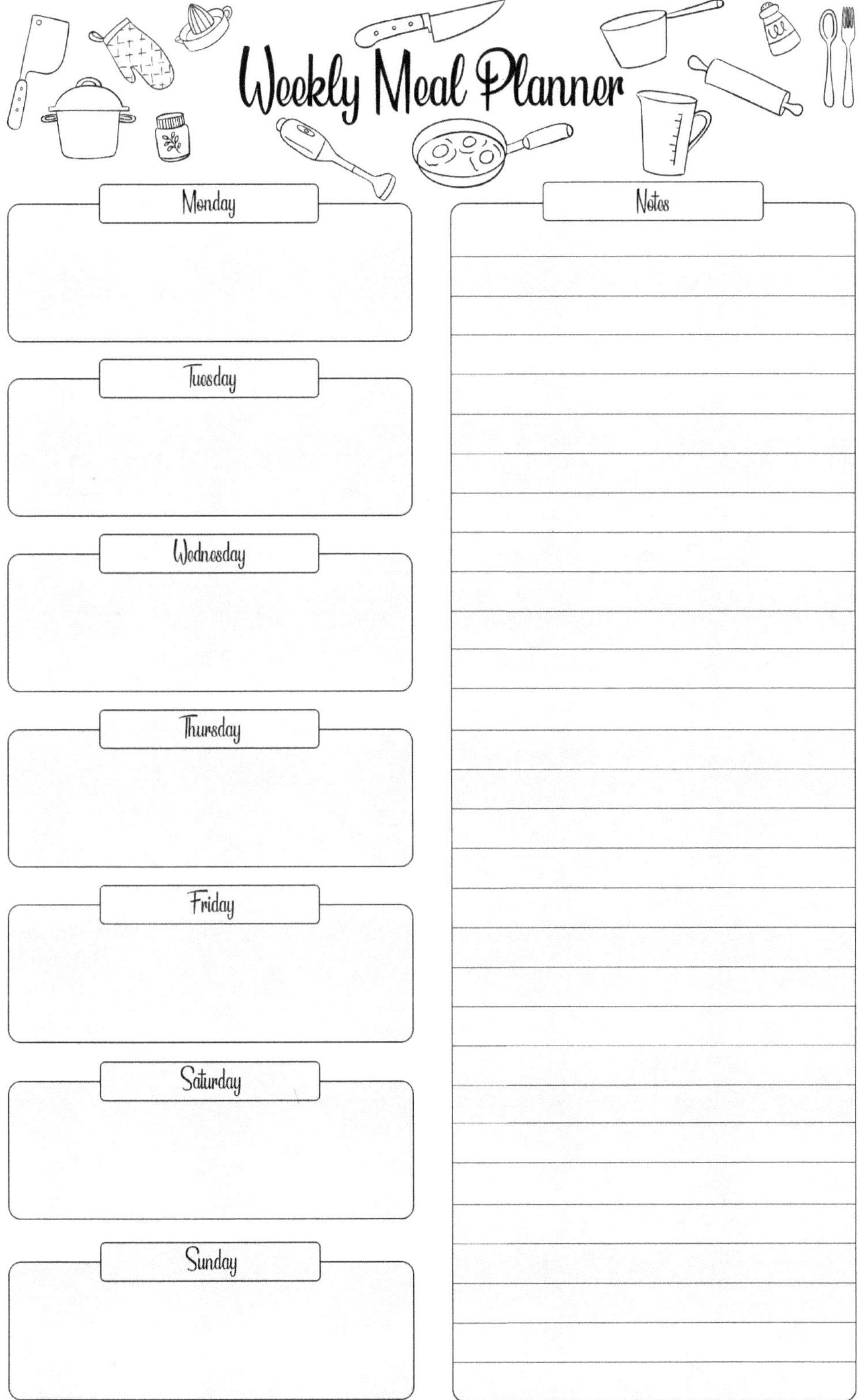

Weekly Meal Planner

Monday

Tuesday

Wednesday

Thursday

Friday

Saturday

Sunday

Notes

Weekly Meal Planner

Monday

Tuesday

Wednesday

Thursday

Friday

Saturday

Sunday

Notes

Weekly Meal Planner

Monday

Tuesday

Wednesday

Thursday

Friday

Saturday

Sunday

Notes

Weekly Meal Planner

Monday

Tuesday

Wednesday

Thursday

Friday

Saturday

Sunday

Notes

Weekly Meal Planner

Monday

Tuesday

Wednesday

Thursday

Friday

Saturday

Sunday

Notes

Weekly Meal Planner

Monday

Tuesday

Wednesday

Thursday

Friday

Saturday

Sunday

Notes

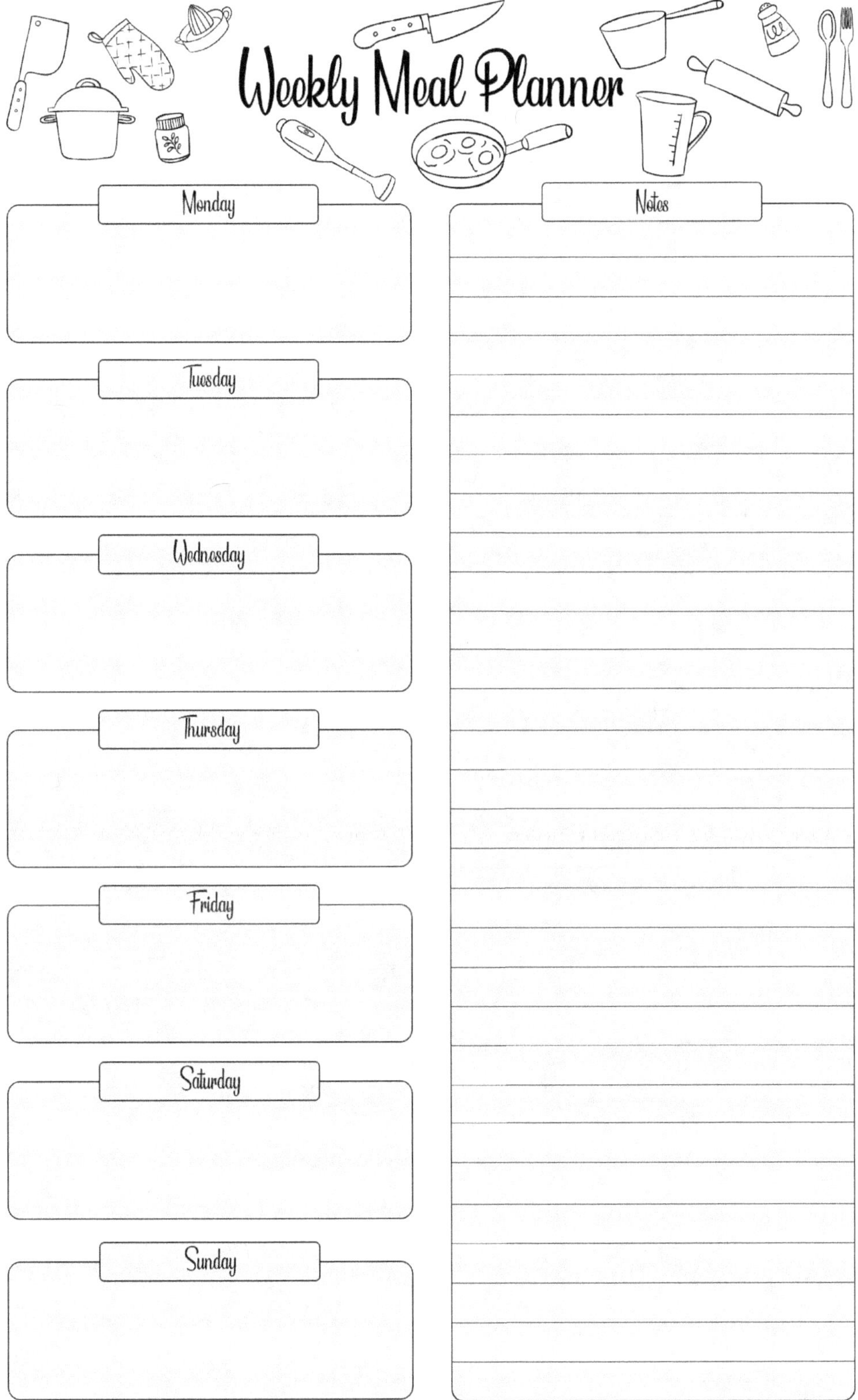

Weekly Meal Planner

Monday	**Notes**
Tuesday	
Wednesday	
Thursday	
Friday	
Saturday	
Sunday	

Weekly Meal Planner

Monday

Tuesday

Wednesday

Thursday

Friday

Saturday

Sunday

Notes

Weekly Meal Planner

Monday

Tuesday

Wednesday

Thursday

Friday

Saturday

Sunday

Notes

Weekly Meal Planner

Monday

Tuesday

Wednesday

Thursday

Friday

Saturday

Sunday

Notes

Weekly Meal Planner

Monday

Tuesday

Wednesday

Thursday

Friday

Saturday

Sunday

Notes

Weekly Meal Planner

Monday

Tuesday

Wednesday

Thursday

Friday

Saturday

Sunday

Notes

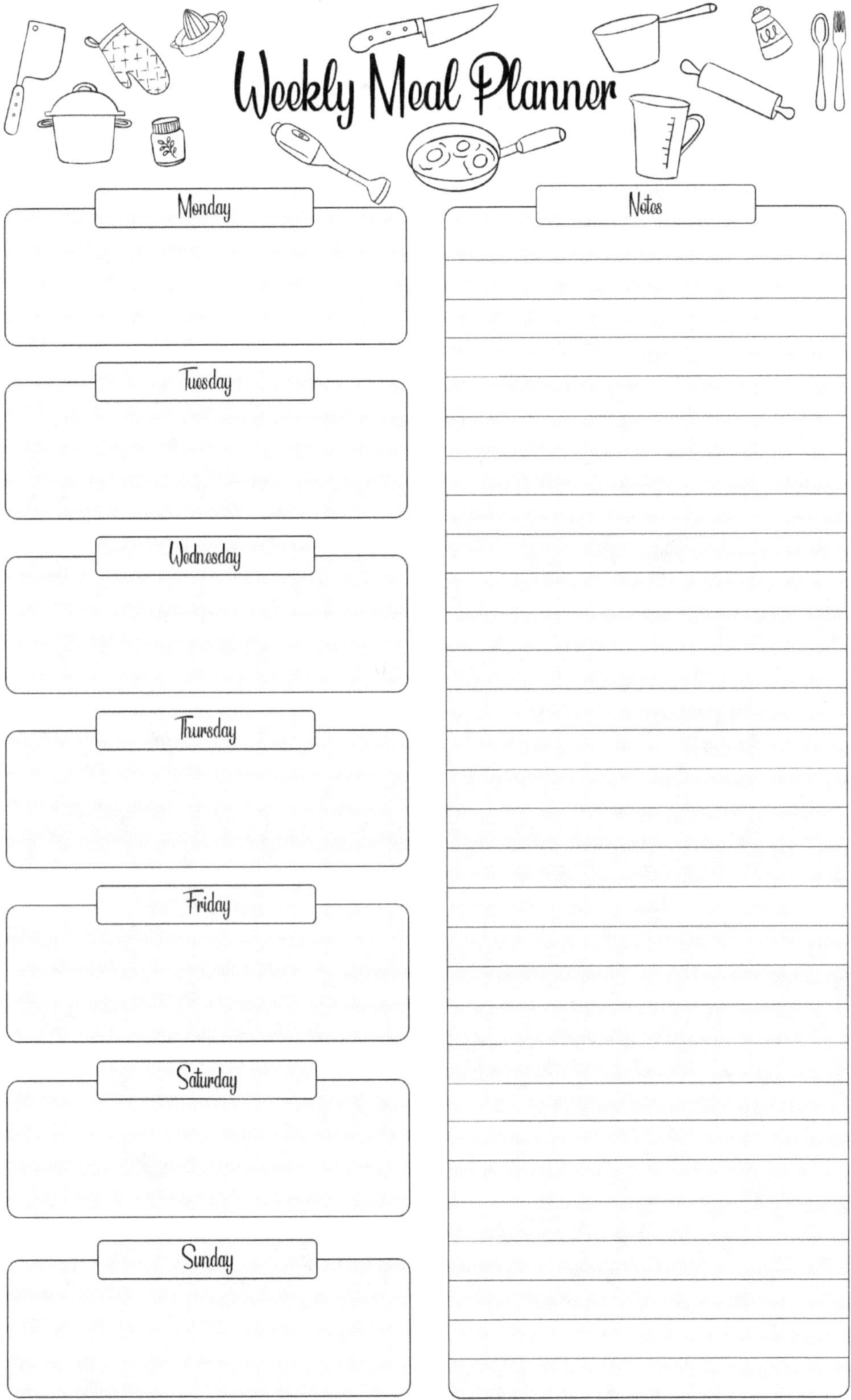# Weekly Meal Planner

Weekly Meal Planner

Monday

Tuesday

Wednesday

Thursday

Friday

Saturday

Sunday

Notes

Weekly Meal Planner

Monday

Tuesday

Wednesday

Thursday

Friday

Saturday

Sunday

Notes

Weekly Meal Planner

Monday

Tuesday

Wednesday

Thursday

Friday

Saturday

Sunday

Notes

Weekly Meal Planner

Monday

Tuesday

Wednesday

Thursday

Friday

Saturday

Sunday

Notes

Weekly Meal Planner

Monday	Notes
Tuesday	
Wednesday	
Thursday	
Friday	
Saturday	
Sunday	

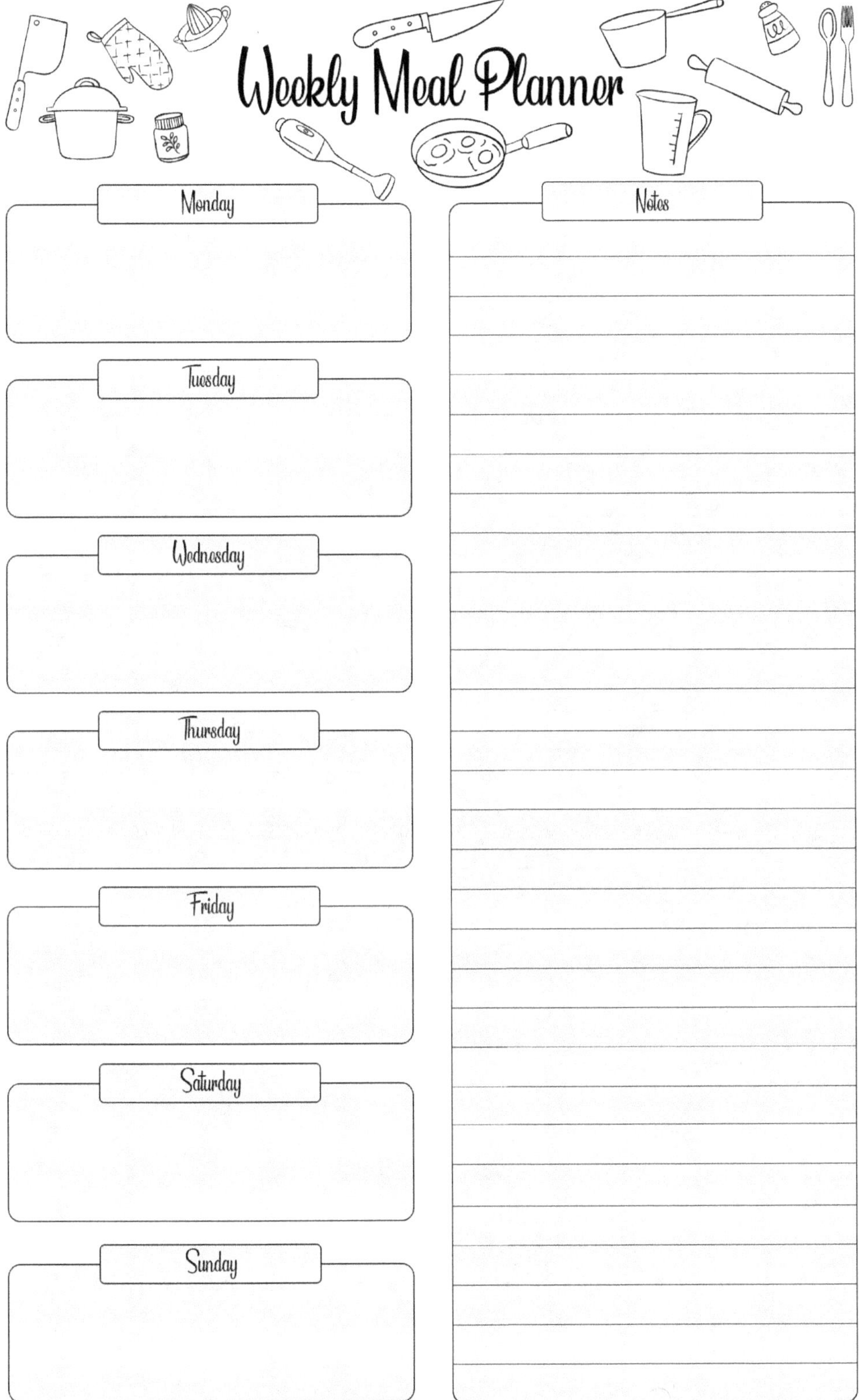

Weekly Meal Planner
Monday
Tuesday
Wednesday
Thursday
Friday
Saturday
Sunday
Notes

Weekly Meal Planner

Monday

Tuesday

Wednesday

Thursday

Friday

Saturday

Sunday

Notes

Weekly Meal Planner

Monday

Tuesday

Wednesday

Thursday

Friday

Saturday

Sunday

Notes

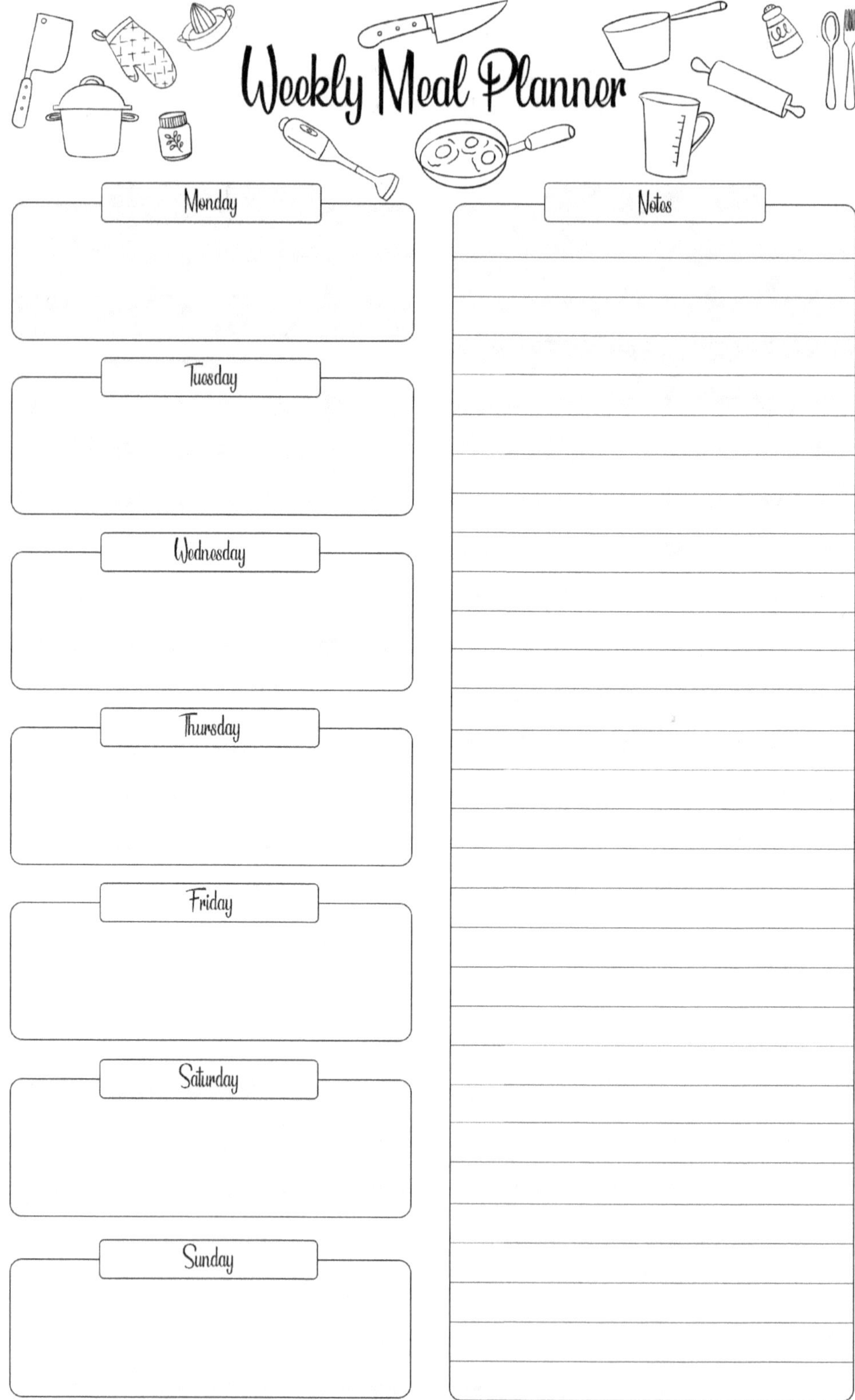

Weekly Meal Planner
Monday
Tuesday
Wednesday
Thursday
Friday
Saturday
Sunday
Notes

Weekly Meal Planner

Monday

Tuesday

Wednesday

Thursday

Friday

Saturday

Sunday

Notes

Weekly Meal Planner

Monday

Tuesday

Wednesday

Thursday

Friday

Saturday

Sunday

Notes

Weekly Meal Planner

Monday

Tuesday

Wednesday

Thursday

Friday

Saturday

Sunday

Notes

Weekly Meal Planner

Monday

Tuesday

Wednesday

Thursday

Friday

Saturday

Sunday

Notes

Weekly Meal Planner

Monday

Tuesday

Wednesday

Thursday

Friday

Saturday

Sunday

Notes

Weekly Meal Planner

| Monday |
| Tuesday |
| Wednesday |
| Thursday |
| Friday |
| Saturday |
| Sunday |

Notes

Weekly Meal Planner

Monday

Tuesday

Wednesday

Thursday

Friday

Saturday

Sunday

Notes

Weekly Meal Planner

Monday

Tuesday

Wednesday

Thursday

Friday

Saturday

Sunday

Notes

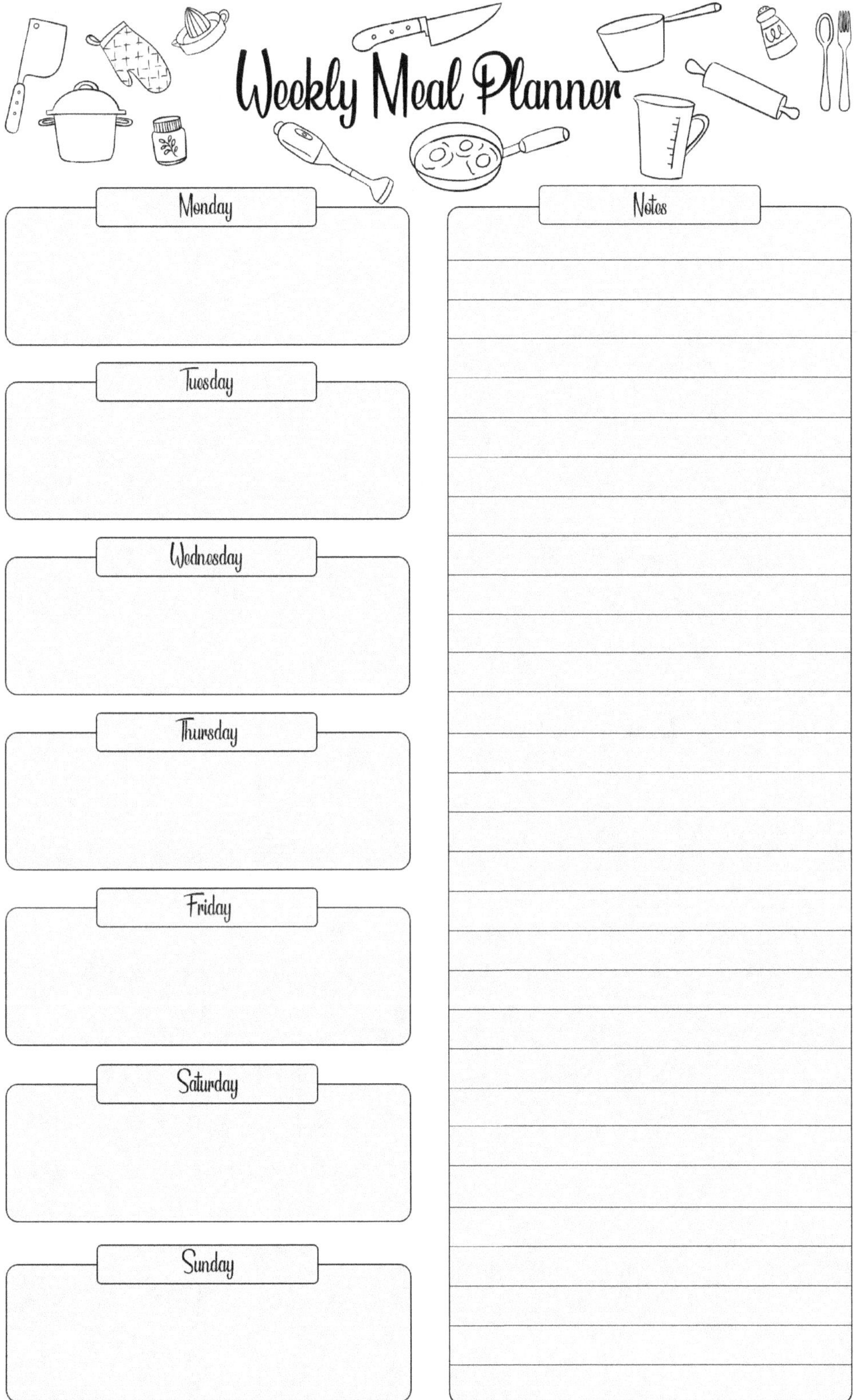

Weekly Meal Planner
Monday
Tuesday
Wednesday
Thursday
Friday
Saturday
Sunday
Notes

Weekly Meal Planner

Monday

Tuesday

Wednesday

Thursday

Friday

Saturday

Sunday

Notes

Weekly Meal Planner

Monday

Tuesday

Wednesday

Thursday

Friday

Saturday

Sunday

Notes

Weekly Meal Planner

Monday

Tuesday

Wednesday

Thursday

Friday

Saturday

Sunday

Notes

Weekly Meal Planner

Monday	Notes
Tuesday	
Wednesday	
Thursday	
Friday	
Saturday	
Sunday	

Weekly Meal Planner

Monday

Tuesday

Wednesday

Thursday

Friday

Saturday

Sunday

Notes

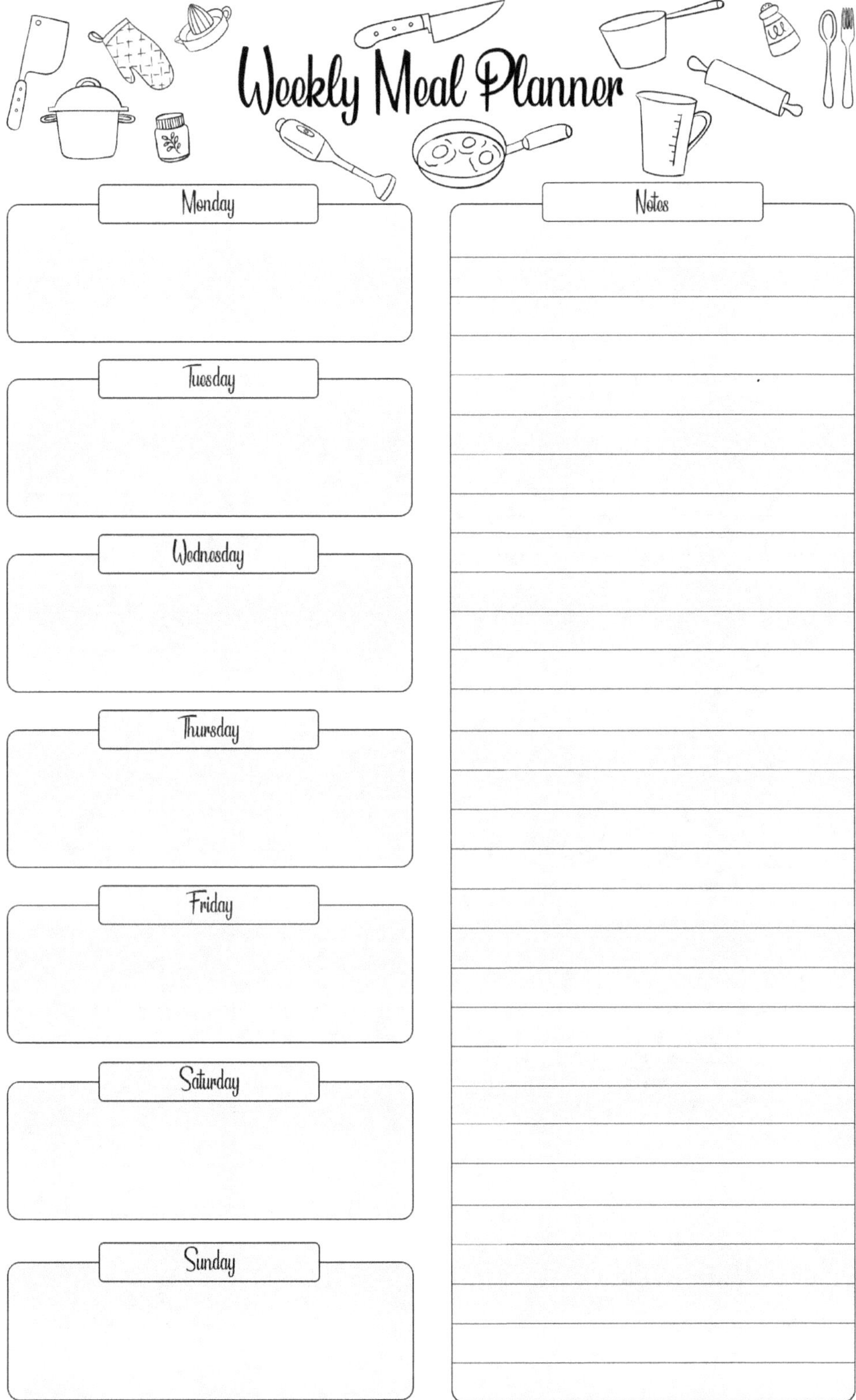

Weekly Meal Planner

Monday

Tuesday

Wednesday

Thursday

Friday

Saturday

Sunday

Notes

Weekly Meal Planner

Monday

Tuesday

Wednesday

Thursday

Friday

Saturday

Sunday

Notes

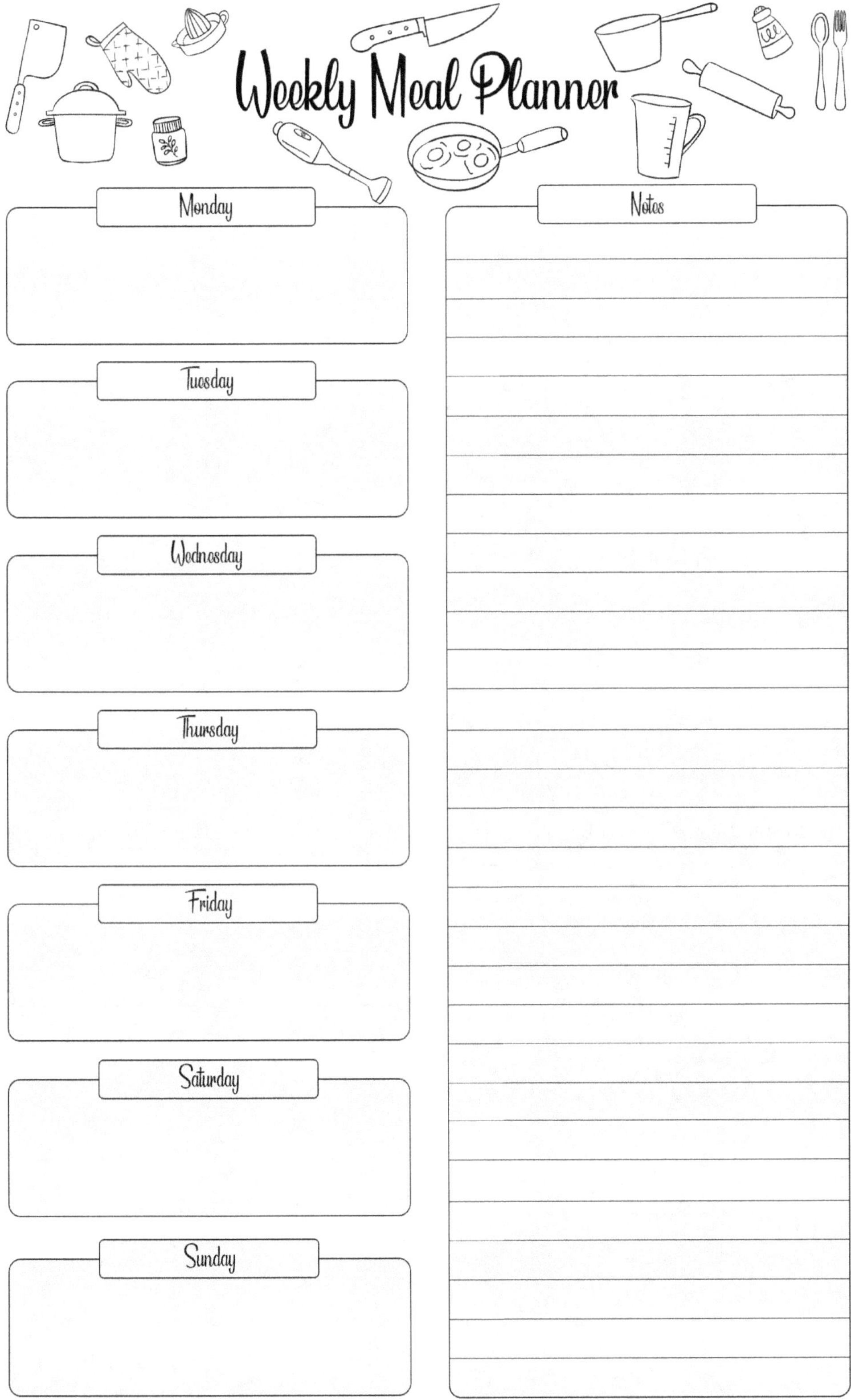

Weekly Meal Planner
Monday
Tuesday
Wednesday
Thursday
Friday
Saturday
Sunday
Notes

Weekly Meal Planner

Monday

Tuesday

Wednesday

Thursday

Friday

Saturday

Sunday

Notes

Weekly Meal Planner

Monday

Tuesday

Wednesday

Thursday

Friday

Saturday

Sunday

Notes

Weekly Meal Planner

Monday

Tuesday

Wednesday

Thursday

Friday

Saturday

Sunday

Notes

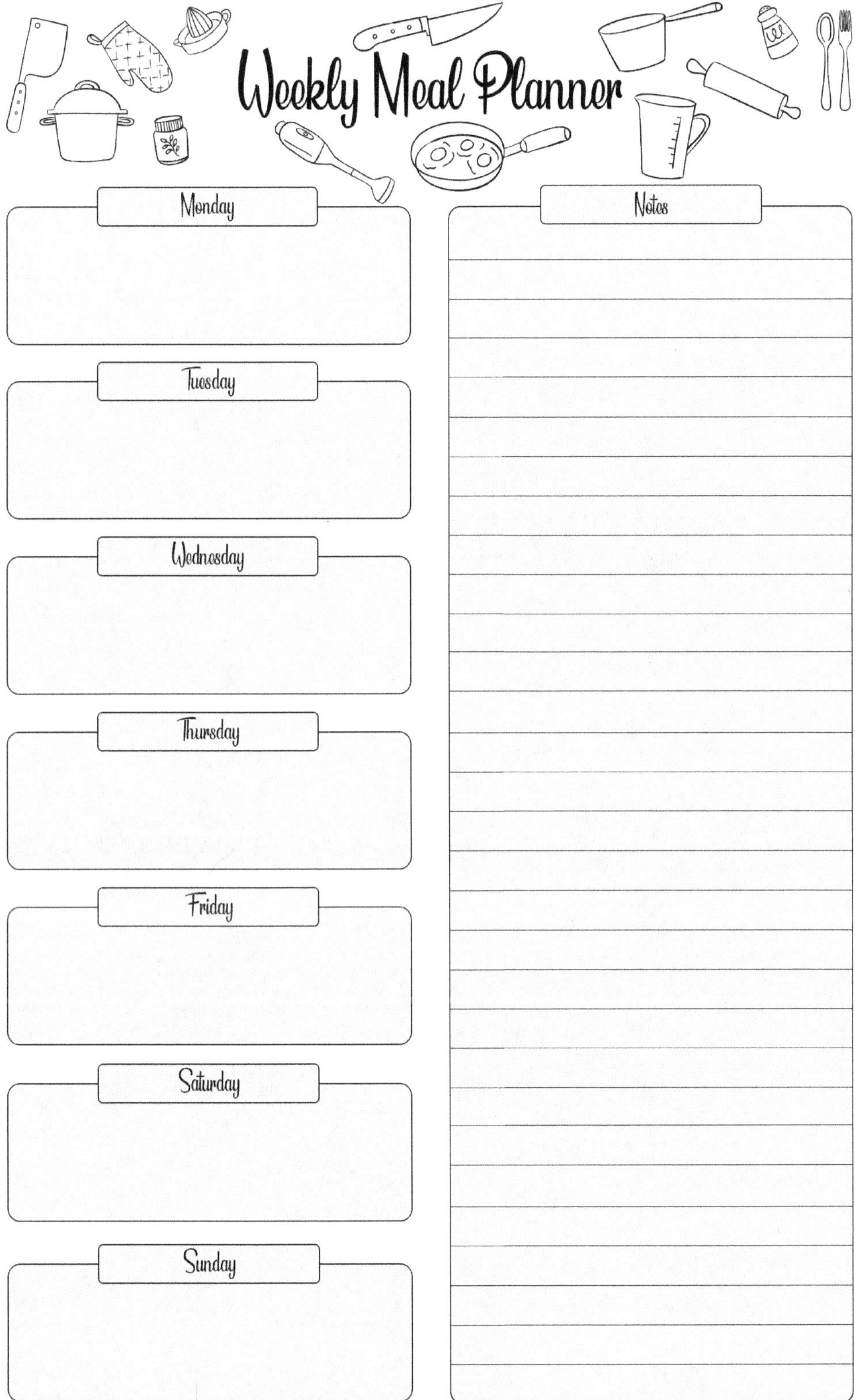

Weekly Meal Planner
Monday
Tuesday
Wednesday
Thursday
Friday
Saturday
Sunday
Notes

Weekly Meal Planner

Monday

Tuesday

Wednesday

Thursday

Friday

Saturday

Sunday

Notes

Weekly Meal Planner

Monday

Tuesday

Wednesday

Thursday

Friday

Saturday

Sunday

Notes

Weekly Meal Planner

Monday

Tuesday

Wednesday

Thursday

Friday

Saturday

Sunday

Notes

Weekly Meal Planner

Monday

Tuesday

Wednesday

Thursday

Friday

Saturday

Sunday

Notes

Weekly Meal Planner

Monday

Tuesday

Wednesday

Thursday

Friday

Saturday

Sunday

Notes

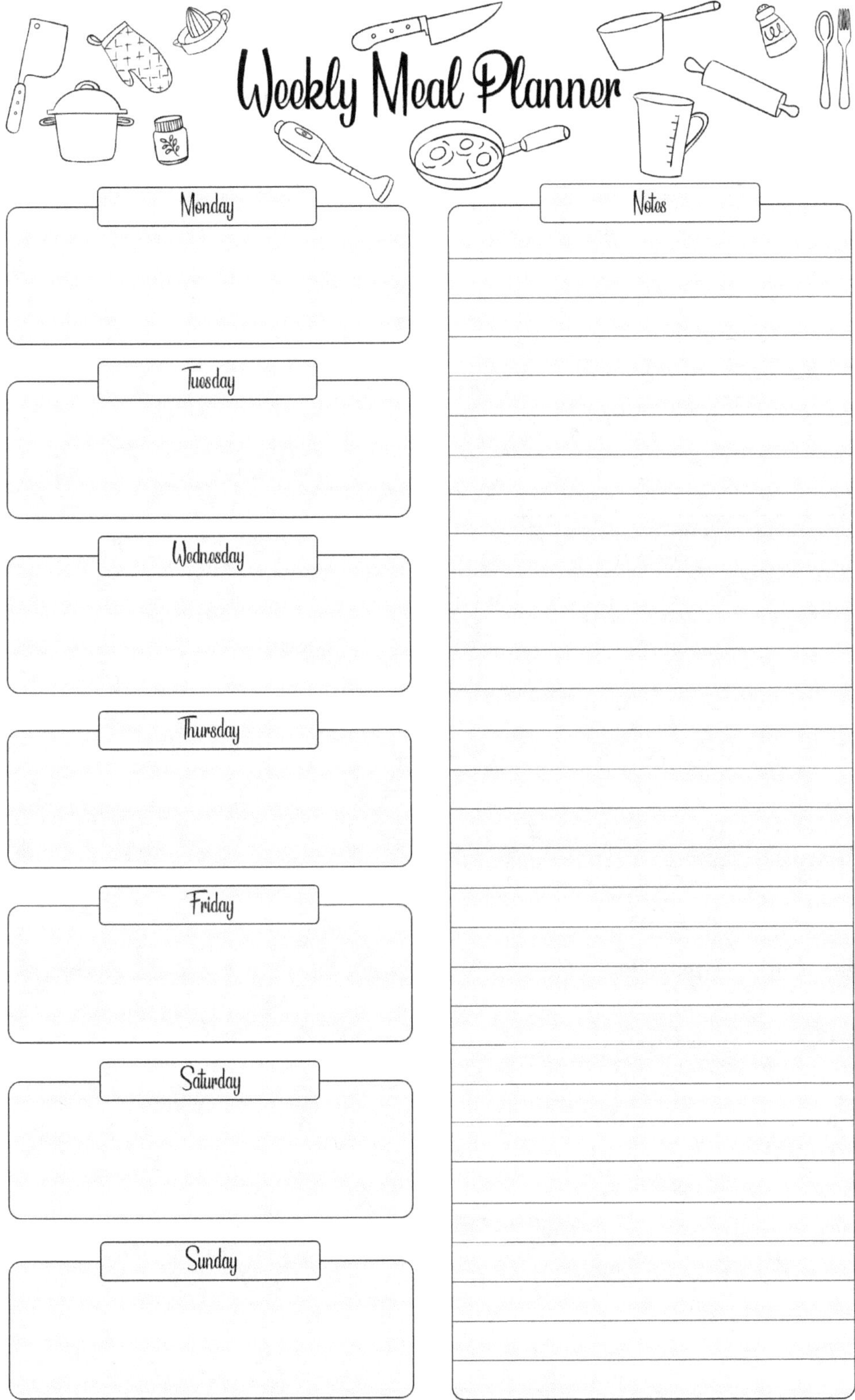

Weekly Meal Planner
Monday
Tuesday
Wednesday
Thursday
Friday
Saturday
Sunday
Notes

Weekly Meal Planner

Monday

Tuesday

Wednesday

Thursday

Friday

Saturday

Sunday

Notes

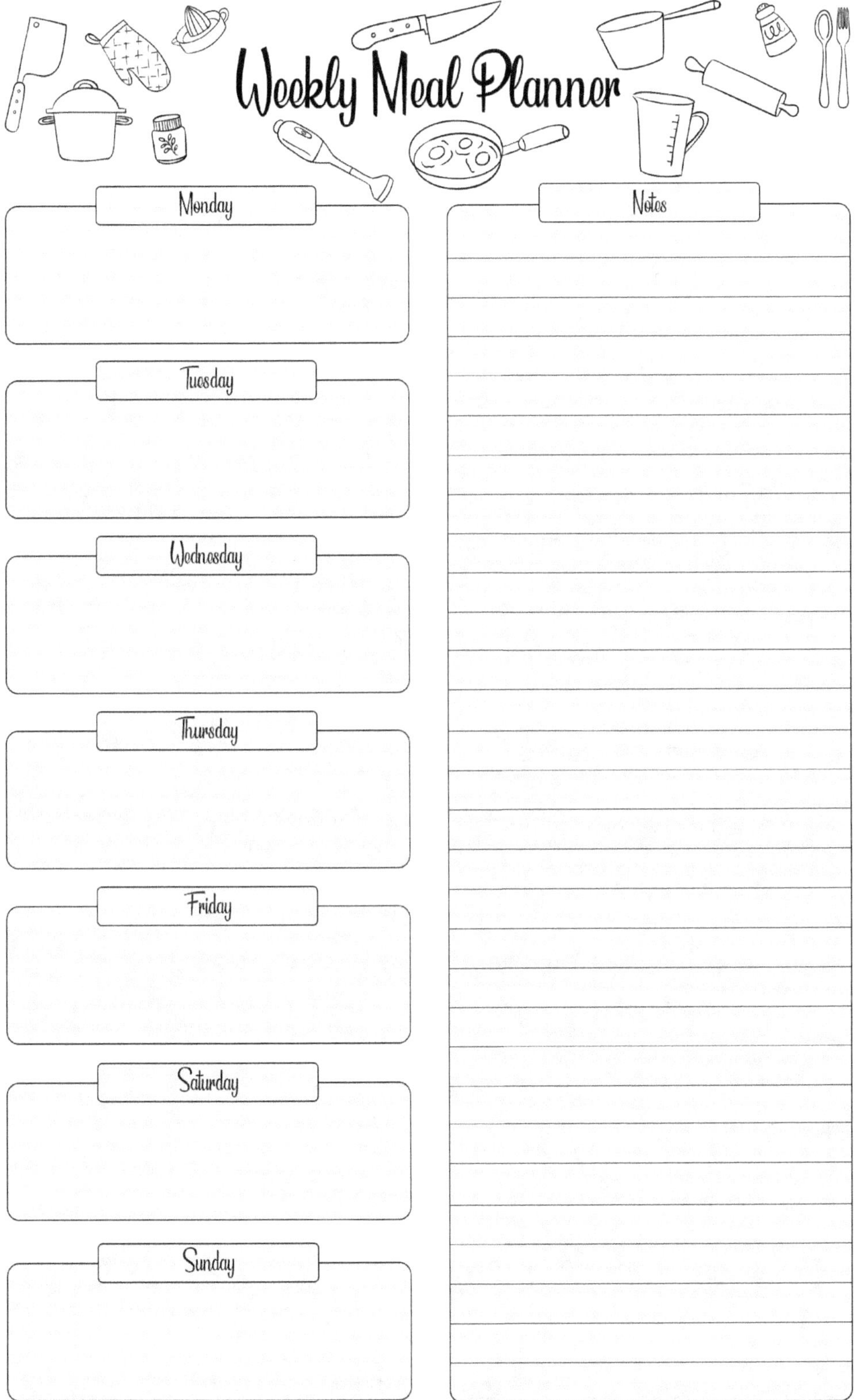

Weekly Meal Planner

Monday

Tuesday

Wednesday

Thursday

Friday

Saturday

Sunday

Notes

Weekly Meal Planner

Monday

Tuesday

Wednesday

Thursday

Friday

Saturday

Sunday

Notes

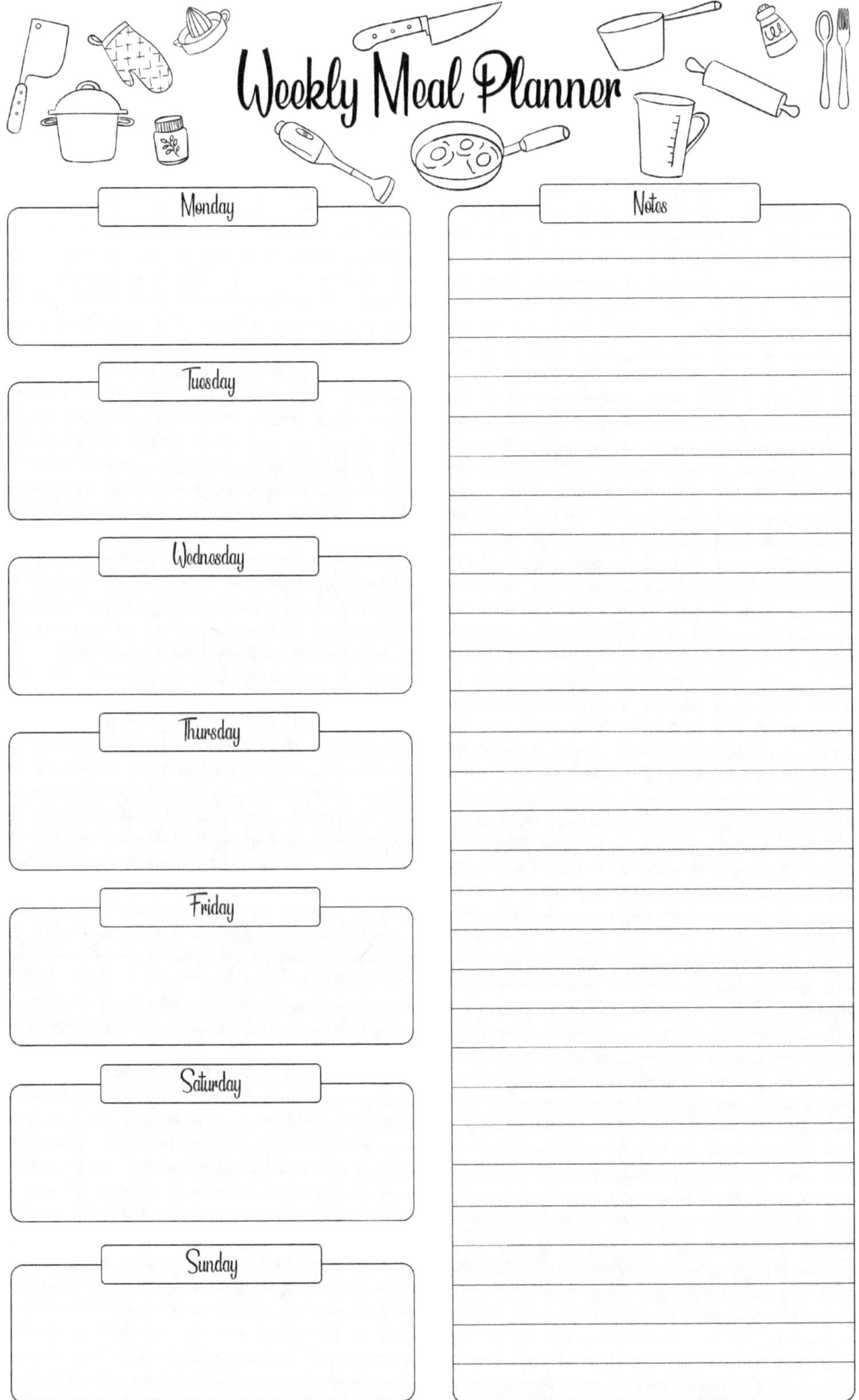

Weekly Meal Planner

| Monday |
| Tuesday |
| Wednesday |
| Thursday |
| Friday |
| Saturday |
| Sunday |

| Notes |

Weekly Meal Planner

Monday

Tuesday

Wednesday

Thursday

Friday

Saturday

Sunday

Notes

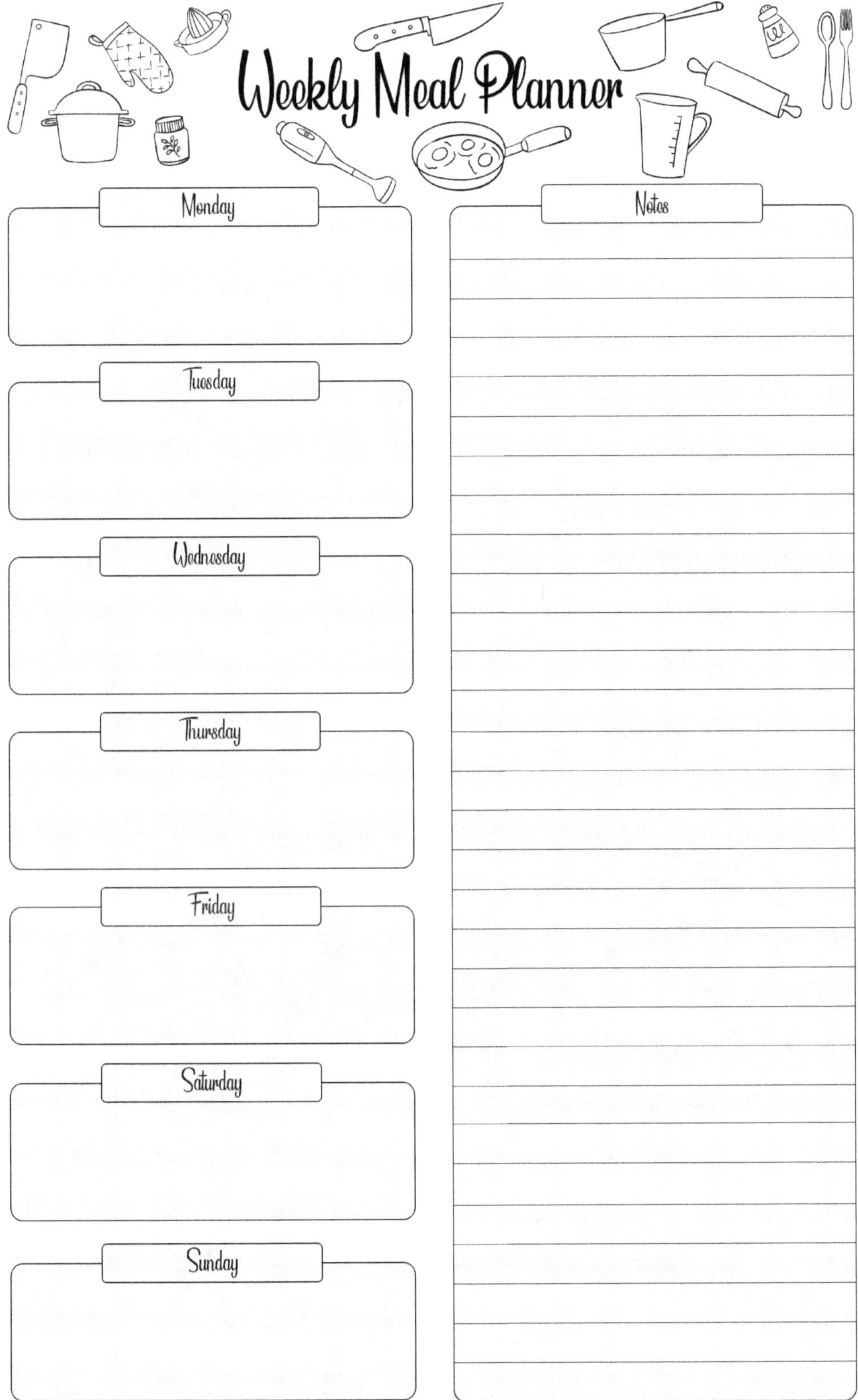
Weekly Meal Planner
Monday
Tuesday
Wednesday
Thursday
Friday
Saturday
Sunday
Notes

Weekly Meal Planner

Monday

Tuesday

Wednesday

Thursday

Friday

Saturday

Sunday

Notes

Weekly Meal Planner

Weekly Meal Planner

Monday

Tuesday

Wednesday

Thursday

Friday

Saturday

Sunday

Notes

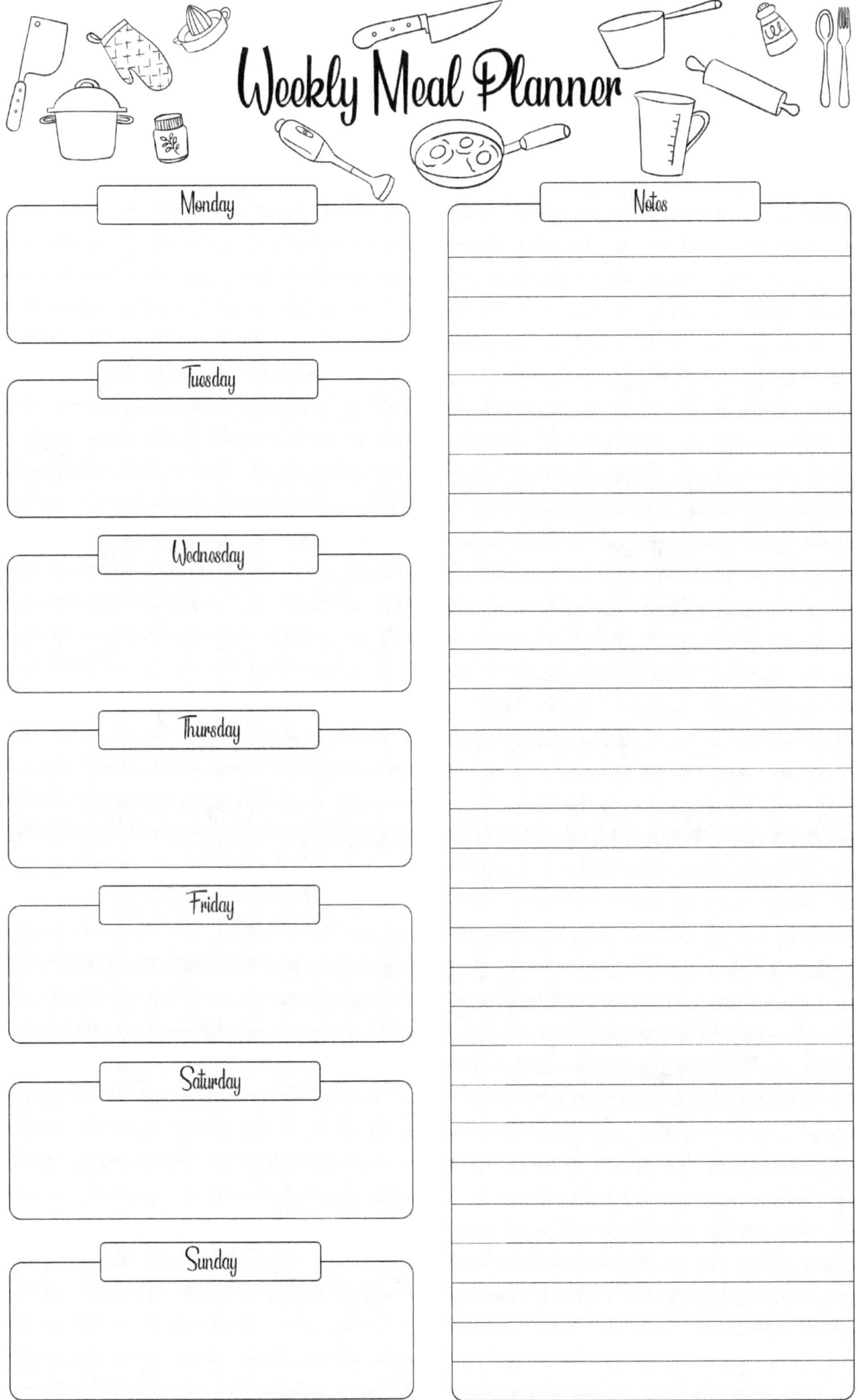

Weekly Meal Planner
Monday
Tuesday
Wednesday
Thursday
Friday
Saturday
Sunday
Notes

Weekly Meal Planner

Monday

Tuesday

Wednesday

Thursday

Friday

Saturday

Sunday

Notes

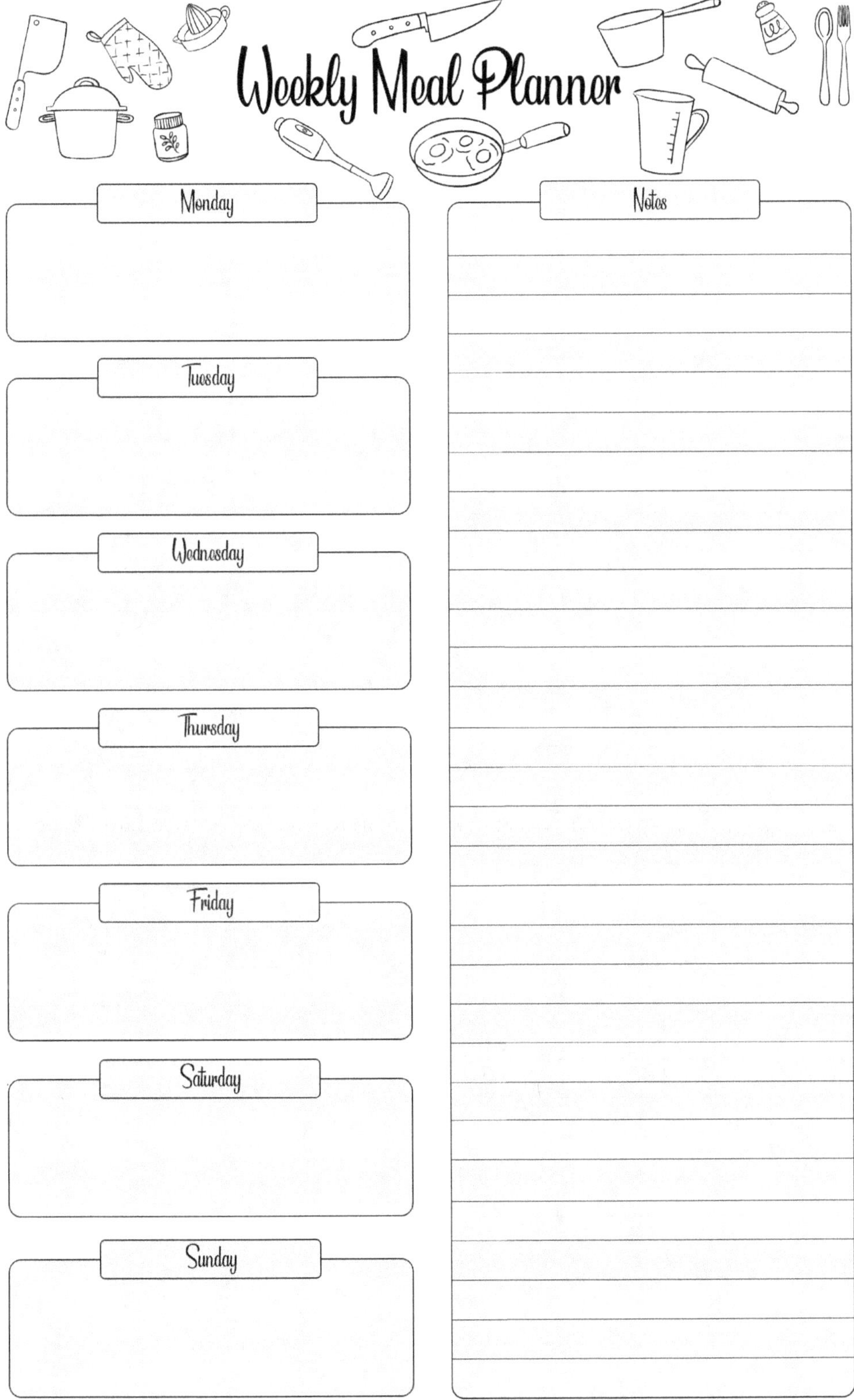

Weekly Meal Planner

Monday

Tuesday

Wednesday

Thursday

Friday

Saturday

Sunday

Notes

Weekly Meal Planner

Monday

Tuesday

Wednesday

Thursday

Friday

Saturday

Sunday

Notes

Weekly Meal Planner

Monday

Tuesday

Wednesday

Thursday

Friday

Saturday

Sunday

Notes

Weekly Meal Planner

Monday

Tuesday

Wednesday

Thursday

Friday

Saturday

Sunday

Notes

Weekly Meal Planner

Monday	Notes

| Tuesday |

| Wednesday |

| Thursday |

| Friday |

| Saturday |

| Sunday |

Weekly Meal Planner

Monday

Tuesday

Wednesday

Thursday

Friday

Saturday

Sunday

Notes

Weekly Meal Planner

Monday

Tuesday

Wednesday

Thursday

Friday

Saturday

Sunday

Notes

Weekly Meal Planner

Monday

Tuesday

Wednesday

Thursday

Friday

Saturday

Sunday

Notes

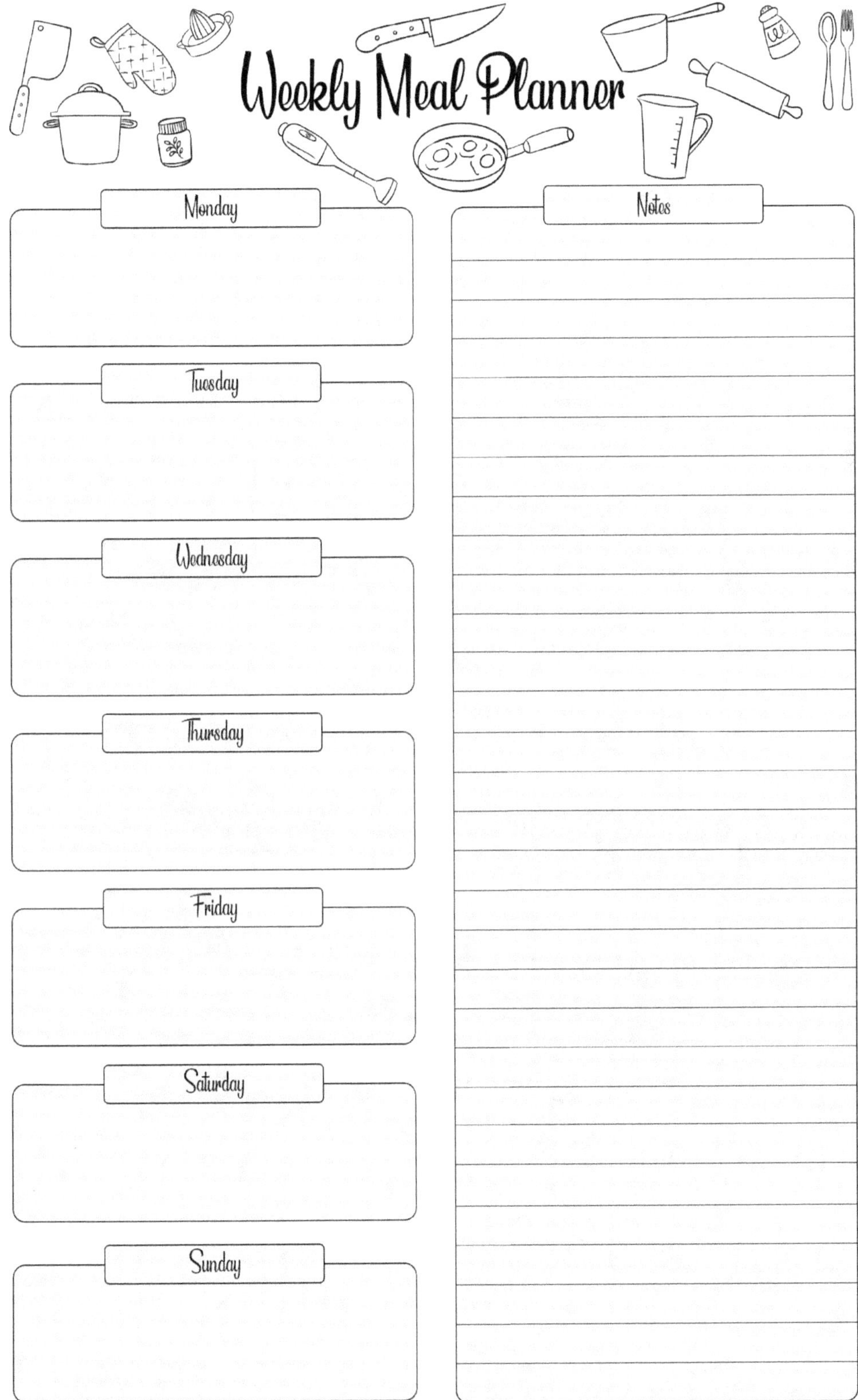

Weekly Meal Planner
Monday
Tuesday
Wednesday
Thursday
Friday
Saturday
Sunday
Notes

Weekly Meal Planner

Monday

Tuesday

Wednesday

Thursday

Friday

Saturday

Sunday

Notes

Weekly Meal Planner

Monday

Tuesday

Wednesday

Thursday

Friday

Saturday

Sunday

Notes

Weekly Meal Planner

Monday

Tuesday

Wednesday

Thursday

Friday

Saturday

Sunday

Notes

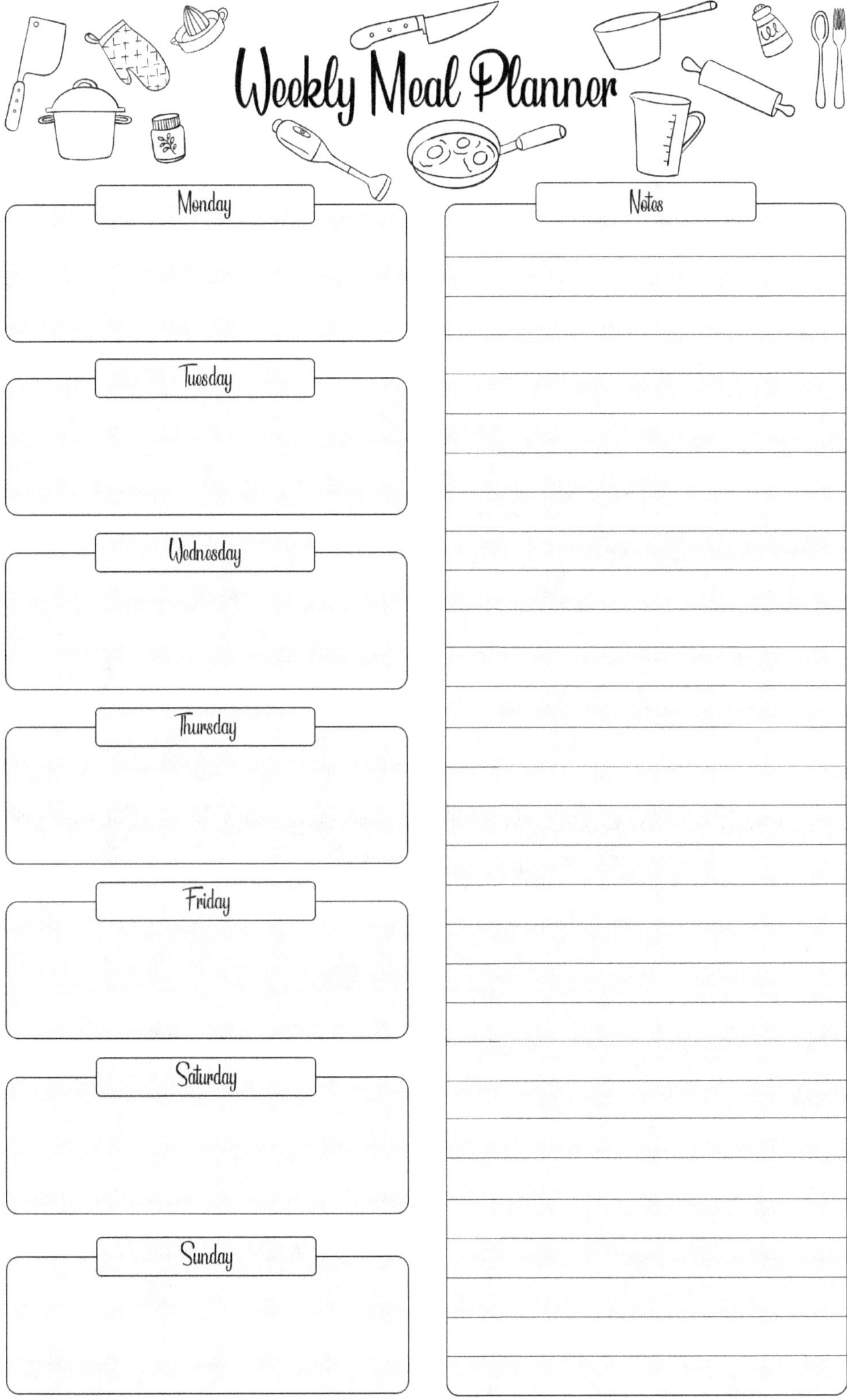

Weekly Meal Planner
Monday
Tuesday
Wednesday
Thursday
Friday
Saturday
Sunday
Notes

Weekly Meal Planner

Monday

Tuesday

Wednesday

Thursday

Friday

Saturday

Sunday

Notes

Weekly Meal Planner

Monday

Tuesday

Wednesday

Thursday

Friday

Saturday

Sunday

Notes

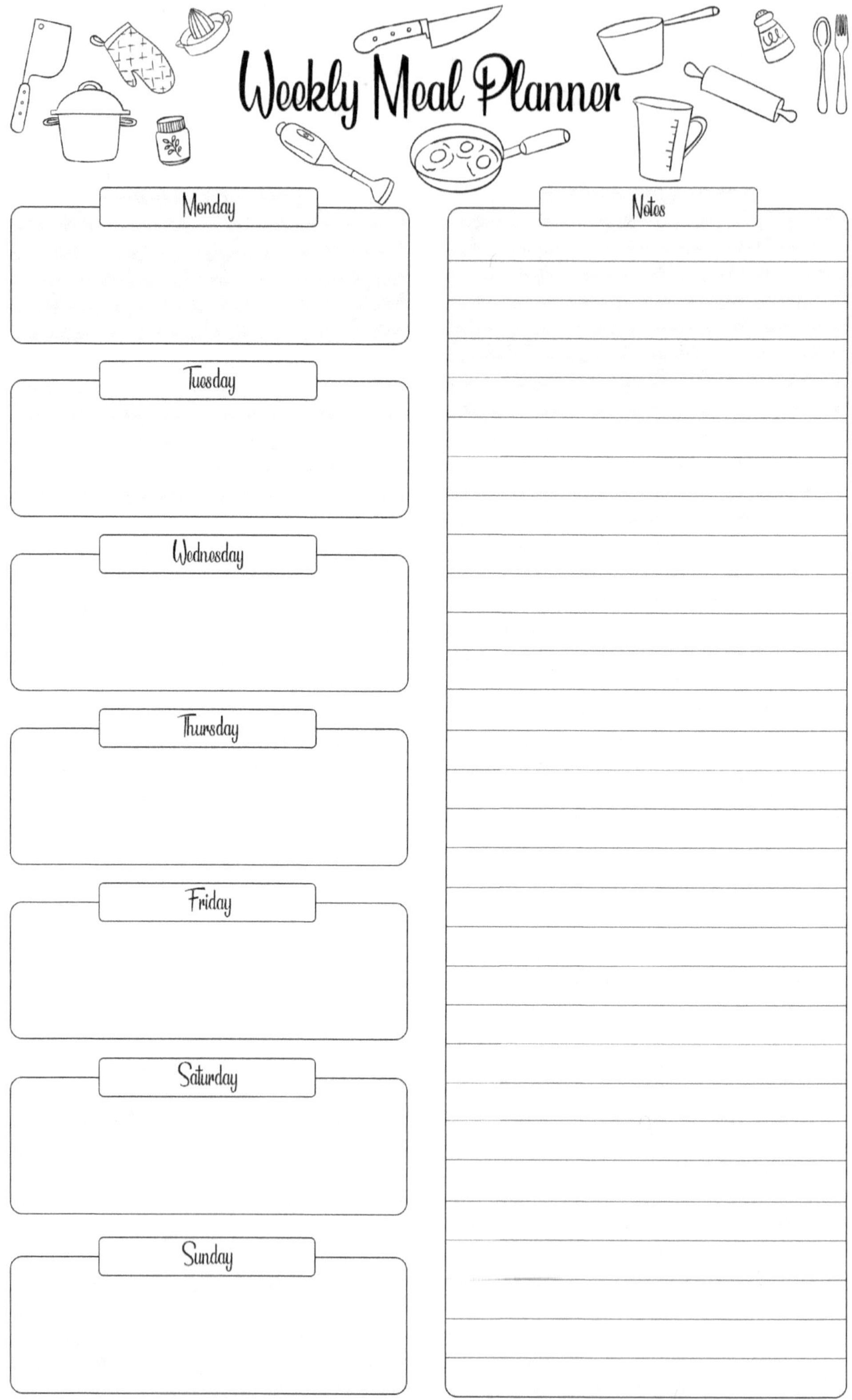

Weekly Meal Planner
Monday
Tuesday
Wednesday
Thursday
Friday
Saturday
Sunday
Notes

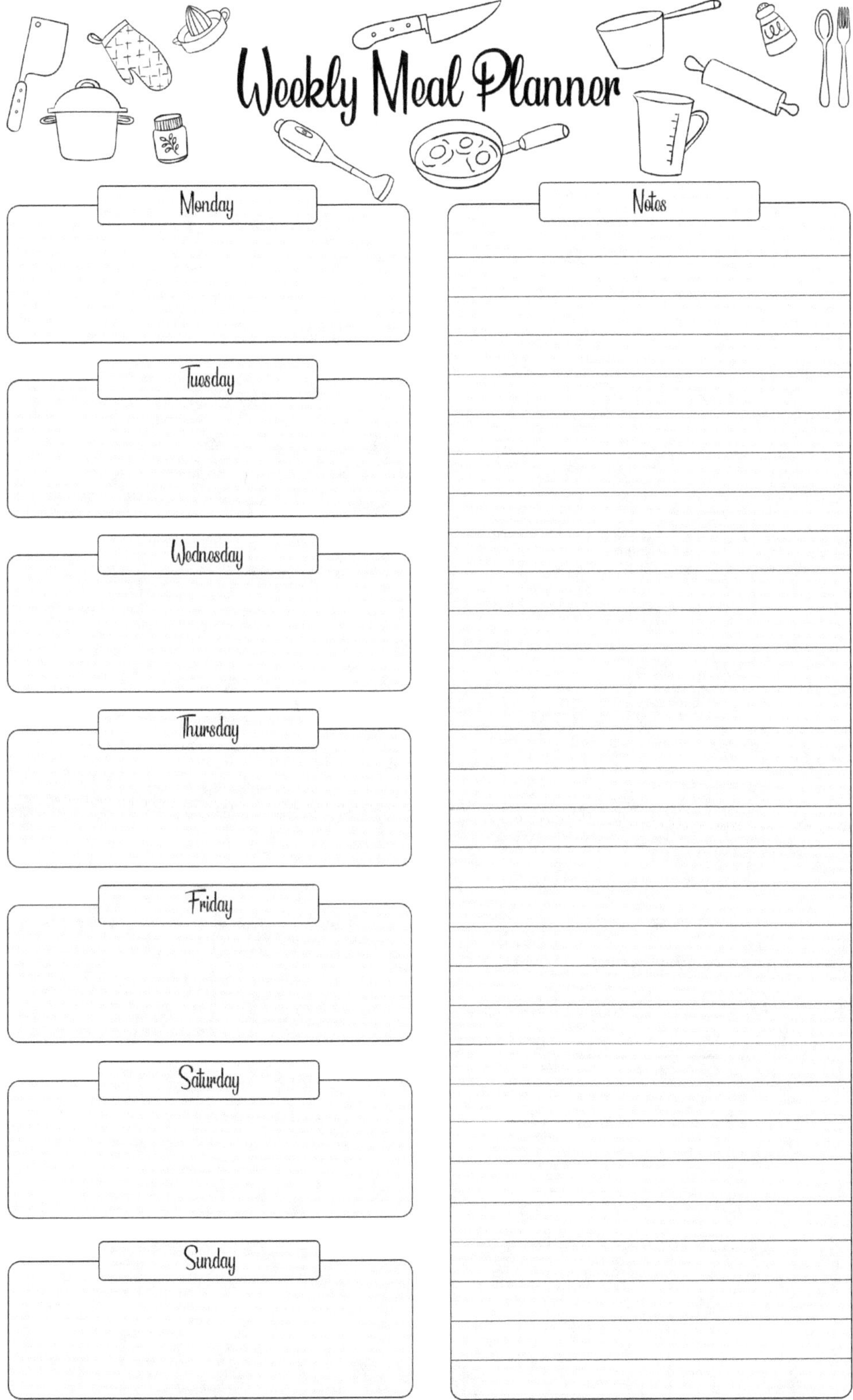

Weekly Meal Planner
Monday
Tuesday
Wednesday
Thursday
Friday
Saturday
Sunday
Notes

Weekly Meal Planner

Monday

Tuesday

Wednesday

Thursday

Friday

Saturday

Sunday

Notes

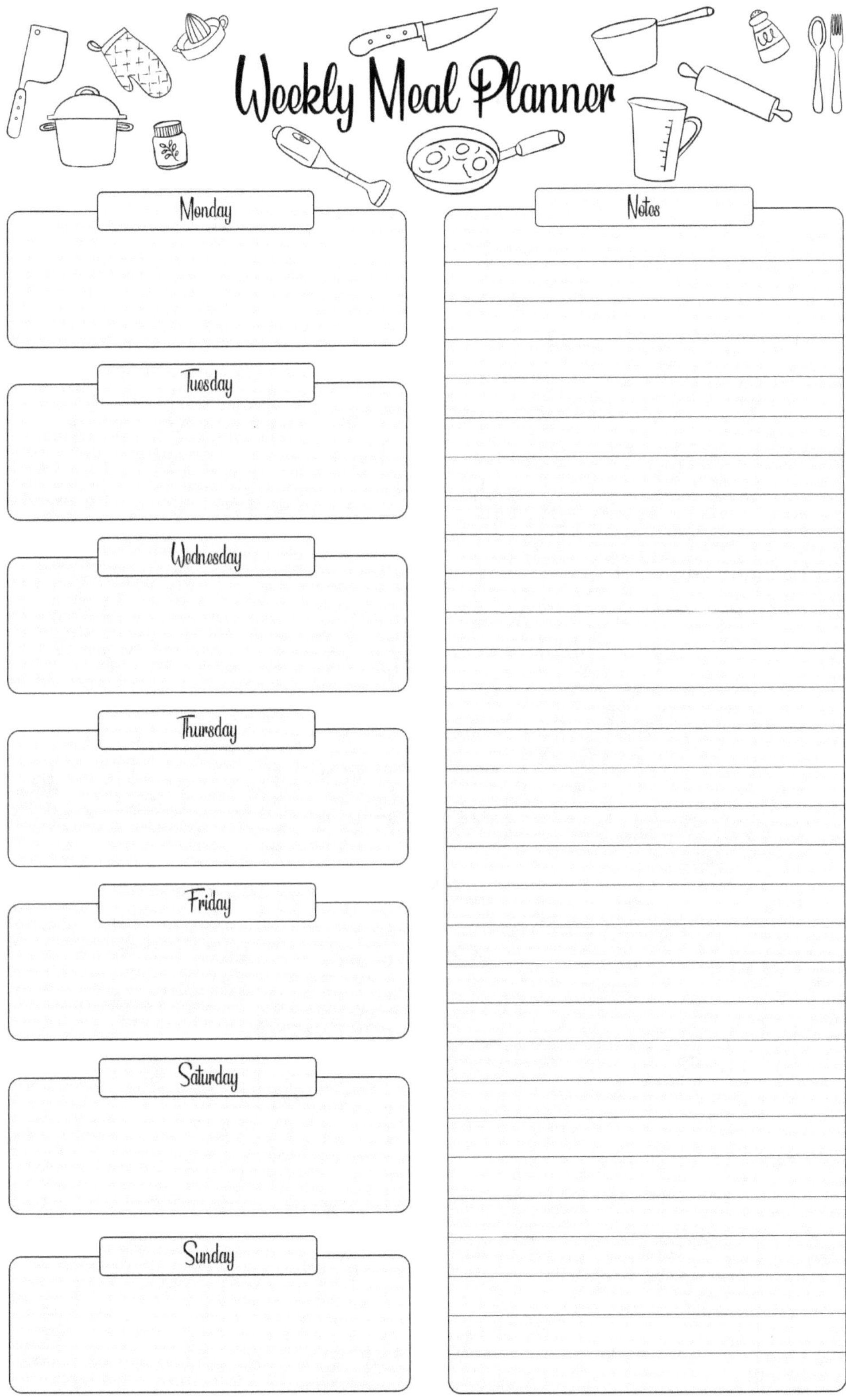

Weekly Meal Planner

Monday

Tuesday

Wednesday

Thursday

Friday

Saturday

Sunday

Notes

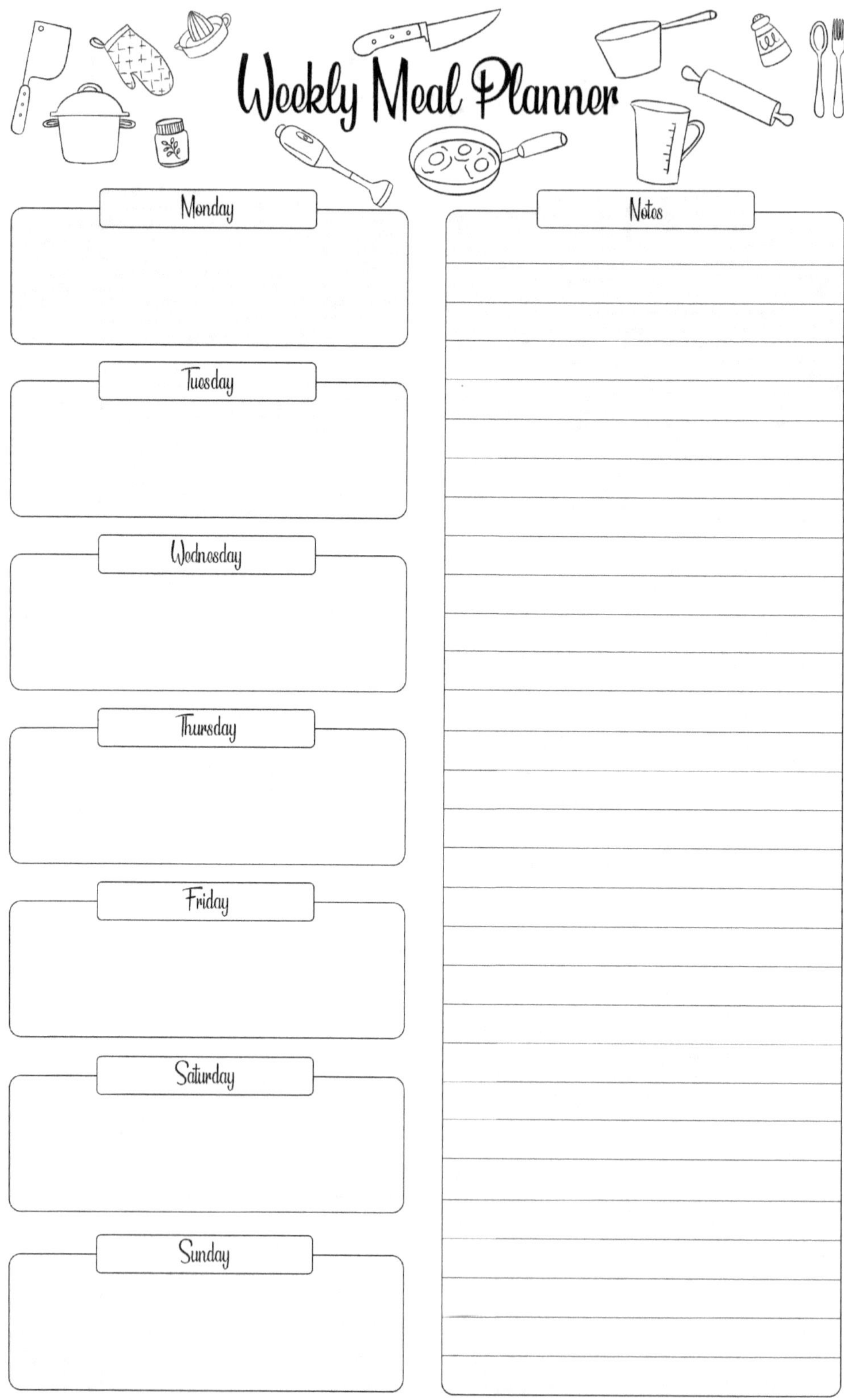

Weekly Meal Planner
Monday
Tuesday
Wednesday
Thursday
Friday
Saturday
Sunday
Notes

Weekly Meal Planner

Monday

Tuesday

Wednesday

Thursday

Friday

Saturday

Sunday

Notes

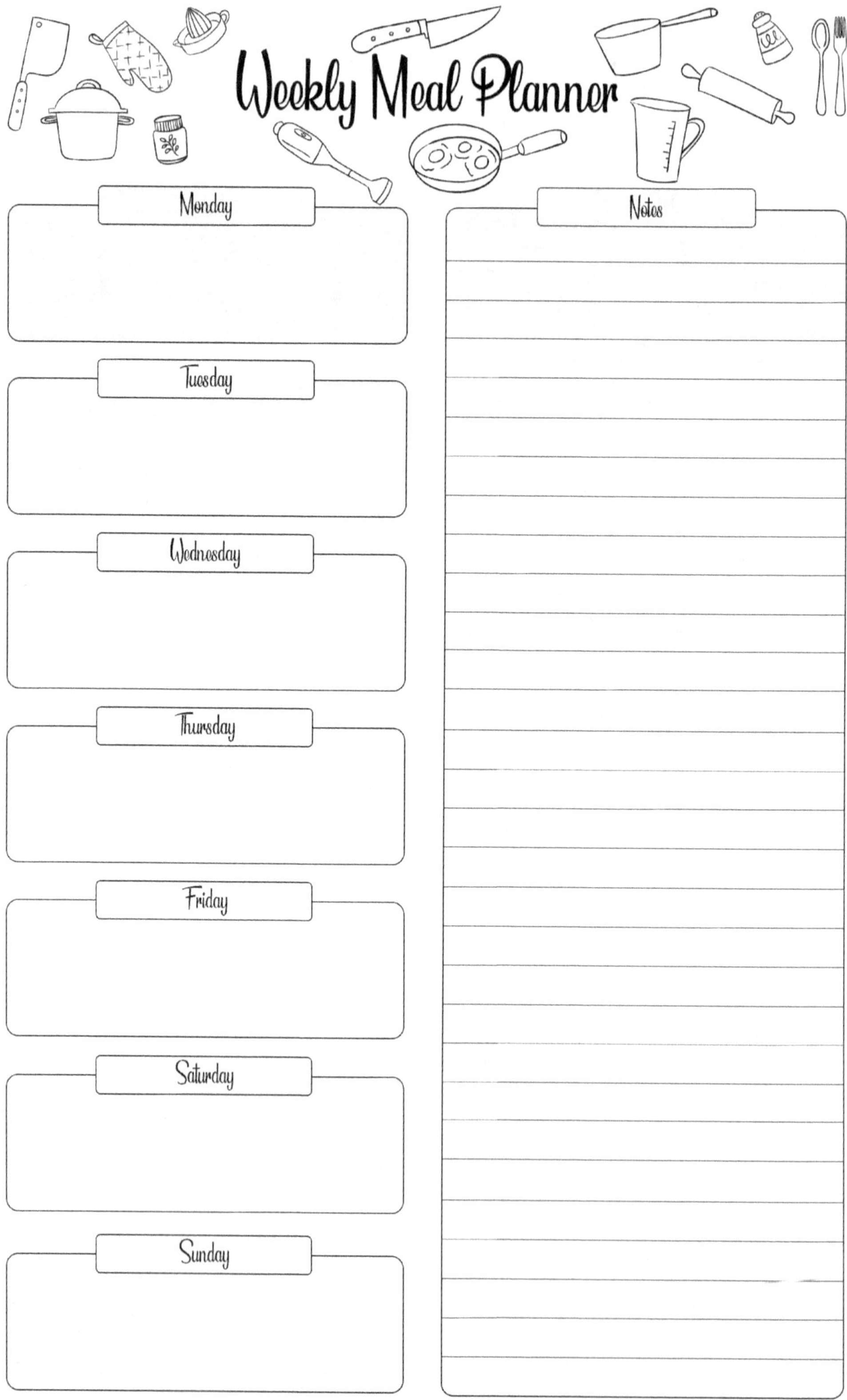

Weekly Meal Planner

Monday

Tuesday

Wednesday

Thursday

Friday

Saturday

Sunday

Notes

Weekly Meal Planner

Monday

Tuesday

Wednesday

Thursday

Friday

Saturday

Sunday

Notes

Weekly Meal Planner

Monday

Tuesday

Wednesday

Thursday

Friday

Saturday

Sunday

Notes

Weekly Meal Planner

| Monday | Notes |

Tuesday

Wednesday

Thursday

Friday

Saturday

Sunday

Weekly Meal Planner

Monday

Tuesday

Wednesday

Thursday

Friday

Saturday

Sunday

Notes

Weekly Meal Planner

Monday

Tuesday

Wednesday

Thursday

Friday

Saturday

Sunday

Notes

Weekly Meal Planner

Monday

Tuesday

Wednesday

Thursday

Friday

Saturday

Sunday

Notes

Weekly Meal Planner

Monday

Tuesday

Wednesday

Thursday

Friday

Saturday

Sunday

Notes

Weekly Meal Planner

Monday

Tuesday

Wednesday

Thursday

Friday

Saturday

Sunday

Notes

Weekly Meal Planner

Monday

Tuesday

Wednesday

Thursday

Friday

Saturday

Sunday

Notes

Weekly Meal Planner

Monday

Tuesday

Wednesday

Thursday

Friday

Saturday

Sunday

Notes